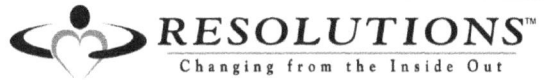

241 Sears Ave. Louisville, KY 40207

Hope Floats
Copyright 2006, Resolutions LLC.

ISBN-13: 978-1467985062
Third Printing May 2006
Cover Design by Naiser Design
Editing by Creative Persuasion
Printed in the United States of America

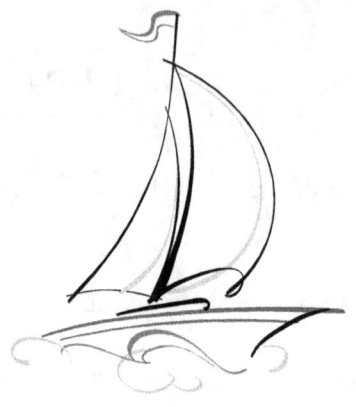

Hope Floats

*Not just surviving, but thriving after **CANCER**
through exercise and eating well.*

By
Greg Ryan
Professional Fitness Expert

Why should you read this book?

Hope Floats is a true story one who dared to dream, to fly like eagles and to refuse to allow others and the voices in her head defeat her. The following pages outline attitudes and activities to help one with cancer not just survive, but THRIVE! You will learn to HOPE again!

Yes Cancer is a terrible disease, but it doesn't have to destroy the spirit, nor does it have to be the end of physical well being. You should read this book if nothing other than to inspire another that there definitely is LIFE after cancer.

About the Author

At age 45, Greg Ryan's career began thirty years ago as a professional fitness trainer. In 1986 he won his first of two Michigan bodybuilding championships. He won his second title in 1988.
In 1990 he moved to Los Angeles California, where his knowledge enthusiasm and skill attracted the attention of fitness guru Kathy Smith.

During this time Greg ran one of the largest personal training businesses in LA. Attracting numerous high profile movies stars such as Brooke Shields, Bridget Fonda, Connie Sellecca and many more. Greg built a reputation for exercise and behavior change and in the fall of 1992 appeared on the Today Show and Good Morning America.

In 1994 Greg returned to college to further his knowledge in Physical Therapy. During this time Greg's gift of motivating individuals led him to production of his own television segment on FOX TV.

1997 Greg relocated to Louisville Kentucky were he built and operated a private clinic specializing in obesity and diabetic weight loss programs. Numerous bodybuilding titles, movie star clients, over a dozen authored books and counting; this has made him one of the most experienced and sought after experts in the business. Today Greg has acquired almost a hundred thousand hours of personal training to go with his well rounded career.

CONTENTS

FROM THE AUTHOR   5
PROLOGUE   9
INTRODUCTION   13

Part I AT THE DOCK

1   Boarding Pass   17
2   All Aboard   21
3   Calm Before the Storm   23

Part II SETTING SAIL

4   Leaving Your Dock   29
5   Setting Sail   31
6   Setting the Course   33
7   Following Your Compass   37
8   Headwinds   45
9   Calming Seas   51

Part III CRUISING

10   Drifting   57
11   Steady as She Goes   59
12   Sailing Winds   61
13   Sea Food   65
14   Watch Out for Mines   75

15   Row, Row, Row Your Boat   81
16   Go with the Current   83

Part IV SHIP MATES

17   Buoys   95
18   Your "Wilson"   97

Part V FULL THROTTLE

19   Full Steam Ahead   103
20   Over the Bounty Waves   105
21   Fellow Sailors   109
22   Sail On, Sailor   113

"Live Like You Were Dyin'"   116
Other Books by Greg Ryan   118
Resolutions Services   120
About the Author   121

From the Author

Two years ago, I decided to parachute out of an airplane. "Why should I be afraid?" I thought, as I looked over at my friend Kathy. She was smiling from ear to ear as she put on her jump suit.

Any challenges in my life seemed insignificant compared to what she had been through. On the outside, everything seemed fine; she always had an upbeat attitude, a great smile and good things to say. On the inside, however, either from the chemotherapy or the cancer itself, things just did not seem the same.

One, two, three, jump! Ten, eight, six thousand feet, pull the cord and then.... silence. Clouds seem to take on a much different meaning when you're above them, looking down. The little irritating things in life don't seem all that important, either.

While I spent less than five minutes total from plane to planet, the experience has given me the lesson of a lifetime:

Hope does float.

Personally, I can't relate to Kathy's struggle, nor do I claim to have walked in the shoes of a cancer patient. What I do know is that choosing to exercise and to eat a healthy diet saved my life, both physically and emotionally. Regular exercise and eating well have been proven to promote better health, even for those who have had cancer. I was lucky - fitness found me. You, on the other hand, must go looking for it.

The doctors will perform your surgery, check for side effects and leftover cancer cells, and then send you home with some brochures for counseling. They do their job well, but there is still much more to do in the days that follow. Survival is just the first step. What if you could choose to have more, to really thrive for the rest of your life?

No, you will never be the same, and most cancer patients just want to return to a life of some normalcy. Exercise and proper eating can help regain your life. It can give you both a physical and emotional boost when you need it the most. It can give you the basis for hope of an even better life, even after cancer.

There are endless lists of physical benefits that exercise and healthy eating can produce; however, it is the positive effects they bring to emotional and mental well-being that really saves lives. Cancer may change your body, but it can't touch your core strengths, your heart and soul. Through exercise and diet, I believe that you have the ability to create both better health and hope for a better life.

Someone once said, *"You can live a month without food. You can live a week without water. You can live five minutes without air, but you cannot live a second without **hope**."*

When times are at their worst, hope is all that you and I have. As you look ahead to your future, have hope that you can regain some sense of control in your life by choosing to exercise and eat well. With these tools, you can continue not only to survive, but to thrive. The question is,

Are you ready to sail?

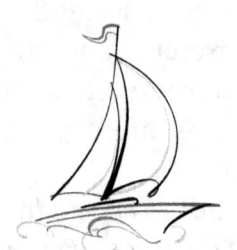

Prologue

We both had done the math. Kelly added it all up and knew she had to let me go. I added it up, and knew that I had lost her, 'cos I was never gonna get off that island. I was gonna die there, totally alone. I was gonna get sick or get injured or something.

The only choice I had, the only thing I could control was when, and how, and where it was going to happen. So, I made a rope and I went up to the summit to hang myself. I had to test it, you know? Of course. You know me. And the weight of the log snapped the limb of the tree, so I...I...I couldn't even kill myself the way I wanted to. I had power over...nothing.

And that's when this feeling came over me, like a warm blanket. I knew, somehow, that I had to stay alive. Somehow, I had to keep breathing, even though there was no reason to hope. And all my logic said that I would never see this place again. So that's what I did. I stayed alive. I kept breathing. And one day my logic was proven all wrong because the tide came in and gave me a sail.

And now, here I am. I'm back. In Memphis, talking to you. I have ice in my glass... and I've lost her all over again. I'm so sad that I don't have Kelly. But I'm so grateful that she was with me on that island. And I know what I have to do now.

I gotta keep breathing. Because tomorrow the sun will rise. Who knows what the tide could bring?

Chuck Noland
Cast Away
Starring Tom Hanks

Dedicated to
Mom and Kathy

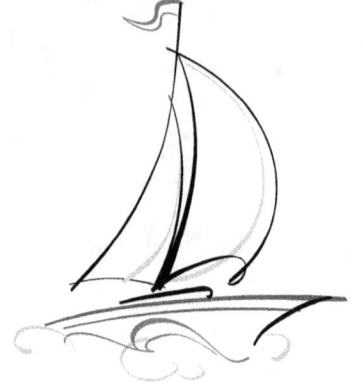

Ready to sail?

Introduction

Life was different now. While on the outside things were seemingly calm, my insides were being tossed like a ship in a hurricane. When I first heard that I had breast cancer, I was shocked, to say the least. Up until then, all my mammograms were normal. I wasn't grossly out of shape and I lived a somewhat normal lifestyle. Logically, why did this happen to me? "Not now, not me," I thought.

The other thing on my mind was "what about my body?" Things were now going to be different on the outside, too. What would I look like? What would others think? And my hair! Never in my life did I think of wearing a wig. After the initial shock, with some reassurance from God, my husband and the doctors, I realized now it was up to me.

Before cancer, I never thought life could change as quickly as it has. One moment I'm going through my everyday items, and next thing I know, a part of me is threatened to be taken away. Maybe even my life. What do I do now? Where do I go from here?
How will I cope? Who will be there when I need them most?
Then I realized it all started with me. Was I going to be the victim or the survivor? Was I going to mope around just enough to get by, or was I going to get on with my life?

I decided that I needed to get on board or else my life was going to just wither away. I had to keep breathing. I had to believe there would be life after cancer. Was it tough? Sure it was. It still is. But, I had two choices; get up and walk or stay on the couch and die. Either I eat healthier or continue to scarf down the junk food and feel rotten.

For the last few years, my sail has been up. The wind has taken me to places I never thought possible. I'm healthier, I'm active and I am determined to go on. Do I know where my ship will take me? No. Maybe it's best that way. I do not wish cancer on anyone, but in some crazy way, the cancer opened my eyes to what matters most to me; my faith, my family and my fitness.

I am so thankful I got on board. What about you?

Kathy

Part I

At the Dock

Derive:

To arrive at a reason
To trace the origin
To receive

1
Boarding Pass

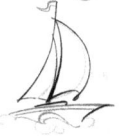

Getting Your Pass

Why, how, when and where? Why me? How did I get here? When did it start? Where do I go from here?

One of the most confusing things in life is when logic doesn't exist in circumstance. All of a sudden, out of nowhere, you get this boarding pass with the word "cancer" written on it. You have no idea which cabin number is yours or where this ship is sailing. Here is where you question your path, purpose and future. What eludes you most is, "Why me?"

"There has to be a reason this has happened to me," you think. In the long run, which question is more important to answer – "why me" or "what can I do right now to start feeling better?"

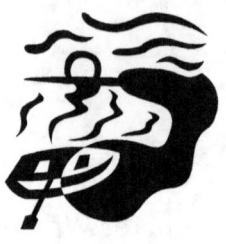

Am I going to beach my life or am I going to sail on?

Getting Down to It

The truth is you may never understand why you got cancer. There are many theories, but you may never know for sure how or why it happened. So where should you focus your energy - on your past or on your future?

Getting Real

The best thing to do is invest in the immediate future by answering these questions:

"Am I going to beach my life or am I going to sail on?"

"Where am I going from here?"

Have you ever noticed how some people get through adversity better than others? Why? It boils down to their attitude. Being resentful or grateful will determine how long you stay stuck on the sandbar. You can stay beached for the rest of your life by being resentful, or you can choose to cruise on out to sea by being grateful for the days to come. Easier said than done, isn't it?

We might just make it. Did that thought ever cross your brain? Well regardless I would rather take my chance out there on the ocean than to stay here and die on this crappy island spending the rest of my life talking to a %&#*@#$$! **volleyball!**

Chuck Noland
"Cast Away"

2
All Aboard

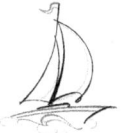

Your Ticket to Better Health

Sailboats and big ships are slow, but they are reliable in getting to their destination. If you really want to feel better, it will take a certain type of slow and steady approach: an *all-aboard attitude*.

Last year, I was on a cruise ship in the Bahamas. It was scheduled to leave port at 4:00 p.m. At dinner that night, we were one table mate short. Apparently, he arrived at the dock five minutes late. Five minutes! His wife said there they were, waving goodbye to each other, and there was nothing they could do about it.

Hey, when the captain says four o'clock, he doesn't mean 4:05. Either you are on board or you aren't.

The bottom line is that you will have good and bad days. So what is the right mindset? I suggest that you buy into this journey, get your ticket and get on board.

Personally, I had no idea where exercise and eating well would take me 20 years ago, but I knew that if I kept at it, one day at a time, fueled by some hope, then something good had to happen. All I asked was, *"God, just give me one more day. Give me the strength to walk today. Allow me to have a good attitude. I'll worry about tomorrow, tomorrow."* Then after a while, my attitude started to change, my health started to change, my life changed. Thank God I got on board early.

Don't be left at the dock - let your commitment be your ticket to a better future. Get on board for *life*.

3
Calm Before the Storm

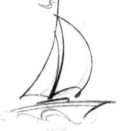

When Time Stands Still

"Mom, how are you feeling today?"

"Oh, ok," she says, as she pats her stomach.

This reminds me of how she would pat my head when I was a little boy and didn't feel so well.

"The doctor says you will be able to go home in a few days."

"Hope so," she whispers as she closes her eyes and falls asleep.

I had never seen my mom in this way. For thirty-five years, I only knew her as the Rock of Gibraltar. But that day, the roles had changed. I was praying for strength, to be there for her.

Mom had colon cancer. *"What? This was just supposed to be routine checkup. How can I have cancer?"*

"Just happened," the doctor said.

"Didn't just happen," she says, whispering in my ear.

Since that day, Mom has lived through two bouts with cancer, first in her colon and later, in her thyroid. Both times, she was treated with successful surgeries and suffered no long-lasting side effects.

She insists that what caused her illness were stress and bad eating habits. Mom claims that in both cases, within two years almost to the month of being diagnosed, she experienced a lot of stress in her life, followed by poor eating habits.

"Didn't just happen!" she says.

I never will forget the look on her face and the feeling I had in my stomach as we heard the doctor say *cancer*. In some way, it felt like time did stand still, and from that moment on, the rush of life just didn't seem as important.

You might have arthritis, high cholesterol or diabetes; these health conditions are serious, but not show-stopping. But *cancer*? What did you do and how did you feel when you heard that word?

Time stood still, didn't it?

First you may go into shock, but soon you start to figure out that you need some sort of coping mechanism to handle the news. So what will you do?

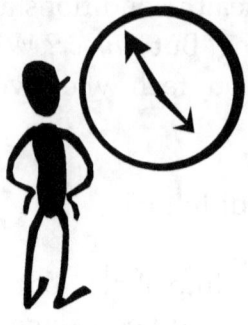

Take time to deliberate, but when the time for action has arrived, stop thinking and go in.

Napoleon Bonaparte
French general & politician (1769 - 1821)

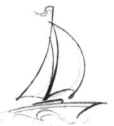

Wind for Your Sails

Hey, life's not fair and when things happen, there is often no logic to be found. So what do you do? You try to accept it the best you can. You get on board.

The goal is not to focus on why, but on what you can do to improve your health.

Yes, the winds of life will come at you from many unexpected directions. Feeling both blown about by its force and numbed by its impact, it may be all you can do to hang on.

First, you survive by just staying above water. Soon after, you're paddling. Before you know it, you're cruising along better than you ever could have imagined. Getting immediate exercise can be the wind that propels you to a healthier horizon. It may be the one thing that gets you off the dock, keeps you afloat and allows you to set sail.

Part II

SETTING SAIL

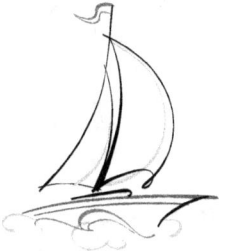

Ahoy, Matey

4
Leaving Your Dock

Fear of the Future

If you are going to sail, you have to leave the
security of your dock. Sure, it's scary to face the
unknown. However, it can't be any worse than
what you have already experienced. The best
thing to do is to concentrate not on the effort, but
on the outcome.

You may think that all of your circumstances,
including your environment and your workout,
have to be perfect in order to start. Such a
universe doesn't exist and it never will. Even in
the best of times, we won't be at 100 percent of
our potential all of the time.

If you want something badly enough, sometimes
you just have to make it happen! By taking
action, you replace fear with a sense of control
over your life.

What is fear? Fear is only:

F alse
E vidence
A ppearing
R eal

Fear of Losing Control

In order to leave your "safe" surrounding of sickness, you have to want to sail so badly in order to feel so much better that you forget your fear and just take a leap of faith.

Having cancer makes you feel like you have no control over your life. At the very least, exercise can allow you to regain some control and to focus on the positive, not the negative.

Setting sail means you have to leave the dock. Leaving your dock is getting control of your life, not losing it.

5
Setting Sail

Wind, Water and Waves

There are many things to get ready before the journey can begin. If you have ever sailed, you know that once the boat is ready, you just untie the ropes, point the bow out to the open water and sail off.

There is such an invigorating feeling about the wind, the waves and the freedom of the water. As you set your course to improve your future, the view of a healthy life, strong bones and more energy on the horizon gives you the strength to make the right choices.

Setting up a game plan can be almost as exciting as doing it. The anticipation of accomplishing something warms the insides. The start of something new rejuvenates the soul. It gives your heart a new lease on life.

One thrill of sailing is being out there on the water and on your way. Nothing can replace that feeling at being one with nature, yourself and your Creator. On your voyage to better health, nothing can replace your determination to do what needs to be done. Where will you go from here? It is up to you to set the course.

6
Setting the Course

The Fitness Attitude

Sailing is more about how you handle the journey than just getting to the next destination. Getting fit demands the same type of attitude. Fitness starts and finishes on the inside. It has just as much to do with the internal, emotional benefits as it does with muscles and bones.

The Right Approach

Let's call this the **"Inside-Out"** approach. My approach to fitness and health differs from that of conventional wisdom. Most programs work on diet and exercise alone. They suggest recipes, calorie-counting books, and exercise tips. While this method may work in the short run, eventually your motivation and desire to get in better shape will disappear.

You have to change your behavior to really make a difference. **There are three things you must learn:**

- What motivates you?
- What are the reasons behind your unwanted behavior?
- What kind of support system is best for you?

The Process

The **"Inside-Out"** approach is not a temporary fix, but is an ongoing process. In theory, it is a simple, common sense idea. In practice, it will take some hope, a little faith in yourself, and lots of patience to master it. The goal is for you to develop a lifestyle that supports this way of long-term thinking. Remember, every journey begins by taking that first step. To be successful, you have to stay on that path every day, from now on.

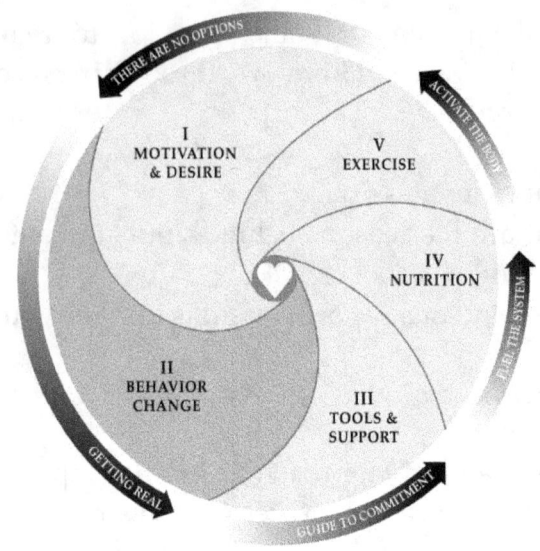

In this illustration, you can see how important each area is in relationship to each other. Becoming aware of your motives and desires helps to build acceptance to behavioral change. Learning about the importance of proper nutrition will feed the appetite for beneficial, balanced eating. Activating your body with exercise promotes long-range success. Success leads to better health.

Each part is necessary in order to make the most out of any health improvement program.

If you have recently experienced your bout with cancer, just try to start moving in the beginning. You can work on changing behaviors later. Let's get physical and the emotional changes will follow.

Those who increase energy levels, strengthened bones, and built up their immune system do so by patiently modifying their thinking and examining their justifications for certain behaviors. Successful living is more about healthy emotions than exercise statistics. Remember that!

7
Following Your Compass

Attitude, Not Numbers

As you can see in the circle, the most important thing to work on is your behavior and your attitude. Sometimes, it's best just to follow your gut. Common sense plays a big part in exercising and eating well. While guidelines are necessary at times, focusing too much on the numbers can set you up for failure.

Don't get too worked up about hitting all the numbers on an exercise chart or menu.

In order to stay motivated, you must have an attitude that always embraces the long-term vision. The narrow view is the futile attempt at achieving perfection by doing everything just right. By keeping an eye on the big picture, i.e. the realistic view of success, you work as consistently as you can, for as long as possible. Don't be a short-timer - be a lifer.

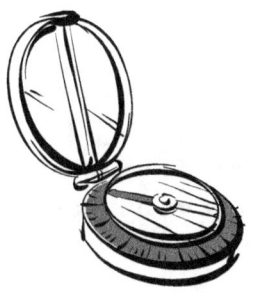

Setting your course is about following your gut!
Greg Ryan

Be Committed for Life!

The military calls them "lifers." These are people who are dedicated to a cause for the rest of their life. Could you be a lifer?

A lifer has a *committed* mindset. He or she understands that there will be discouraging times along with good, and their commitment carries them through them all. You may not be a lifer today, but you could be in time. A good philosophy to have is:

"GOALS CHANGE, DECISIONS DON'T"

This means you must be flexible and focused at the same time. It also means once a decision is made, no matter how hard or long the journey, there is no going back.

Self-motivation

No matter how small, there must the spark of self-motivation to keep the fire going.
The only thing that will get you through this difficult time is to let your hope feed your need for a better life. Your motivation could be fear of getting cancer again or a desire to feel better. Either way, find something to fuel that engine for change.

Self-discipline

Having self-discipline is different than being self-motivated. You can be motivated, but not disciplined.

On the other hand, you can't be disciplined without being motivated. Being self-disciplined requires you to consistently keep your main goal in mind, each step, each day, maybe even each moment at a time!

Knowledge is Power

One of the best attitudes you can have is never to be afraid to ask for help. If you want to feel better, find someone you can trust to meet your needs and get advice. Cancer has a way of pushing aside your pride to make room for emotional growth.
Take advantage of your new self-awareness and connect with those that can help you achieve your goals.

Beliefs

Hope

All it takes to get started is a small amount of hope - hope that you can feel better, lower your stress levels and build up your immune system. At the end of the day, hope will help you feel happier inside and out.

Faith

Sometimes it takes faith from others to get you started. However, the belief that it is possible to feel better gives you motivation to make the changes, keep them going and reach your goals.

Desire

Desire comes from within. It motivates you when you really want to be in denial, be prideful, make excuses or quit. There is no magic; the power to create positive change lies in the passion of your heart.

Formulas

If there was some magic formula to follow, it would have four ingredients: consistency, variety, efficiency and discipline.

Be Consistent

Results are about being consistent and patient. No matter where you start in your activity, the key ingredient is being consistent. If once a week is all you can walk, be consistent.

Being consistent with a small commitment is more important than a bigger effort performed sporadically.

Be Flexible

Your body is very smart and has a keen ability to adapt to things. On occasion, throw a little change in the mix. Make activity fun, but do not make it predictable. Your individual workouts can be less strenuous if you put more variety in your exercise routine.

Be Efficient

Getting more energy, strengthening bones and building up immune systems is more about doing things smarter and less about working harder. Develop a "less is more" attitude and watch the rest follow.

Be Disciplined

Exercising takes discipline and courage. Anything you have ever done in life has taken hard work, perseverance and the will to do what it takes to succeed. If you want to feel better, *you have to be disciplined.*

You must be driven to feel better, beyond the excuses or the self-doubt. You have to be almost desperate to improve yourself. Just experiencing the urge to feel better will not make it easier to start your exercise habits, however. You may have some emotional road blocks to get through first. If you have not been exercising, obviously there has to be a reason.

Your goal is not to resist exercise.

Calm your mind and the rest with follow.

Greg Ryan

8
Headwinds

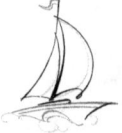

Exercise Resistance

Some people have hang-ups about exercise and food. **"Exercise Resistance"** or ER means a conscious or unconscious block against participating in a regular exercise program. Studies show that people build up barriers due to past experiences that gave them a negative mindset toward exercise and/or food. This prevents them from starting or following through with a fitness program.

ER comes from one or all of these sources: resentment, failure, a desire for perfection, comparison of self to others or expectations that are too high.

Resentment

Have you ever thought like this?
I don't deserve this situation. Why should I have to start exercising now? It won't do any good.

A lack of desire to exercise is one thing, but resentment of the need for exercise to create a better life can be paralyzing. Chronic resentment is much more than just a dislike of the effort it takes to make personal improvements. Long-term resentment perpetuates bad attitudes and feeds stress. Are you resentful because of cancer? You must learn to let go of those negative feelings so that you can move forward with your journey.

Denial

Even if the outside looks good, damage can still be happening on the inside. Over time, you have become comfortable with certain lifestyle habits. You have chosen to overlook the long-term consequences of your behaviors.

Denial is very deceiving. Are you in denial that you need to get in better shape and exercise? Are you in denial of your cancer?

Pride

Maybe you've heard your inner critic say, *"I can't let them see me sweat or show any signs of weakness"* or *"if I can't do it on my own, then I won't do it at all."*

Too much pride costs millions of lives every year. Asking for help may be the biggest obstacle of all. At this point, can you afford the price of pride?

Laziness

Even I have told myself this one, *"I'll start tomorrow on my exercise program."*

Exercise and eating the right foods takes discipline and planning. For some, it seems like too much to ask. Will you give up?

Why is America the most out-of-shape, disease-ridden nation in the world? Denial, pride and laziness! It's really that simple. If you think a pill, surgery or wishful thinking will give you good health, think again.

Denial, pride and laziness can be the end for some, but recognizing these challenges can be the beginning for you. Don't let your mind play tricks with your health. When it comes to developing more positive habits, don't think – just do it!

Failure

Why should I start exercising? I won't follow through – I never have before. It will turn out to be just one more failure.

The real failure is not starting at all. Success is not measured in numbers - it is measured by the growth realized throughout the process. Your "iffy" track record has no bearing on the future of your health. Are you afraid of failing?

Fear of failure is only an excuse to never try. Not making the effort is true failure.

Perfection

Here's that inner critic again, *"Why can't I do this the way I know I should? I might as well not do anything if I can't do it right."*

If you think that you are going to be perfect in sticking to an exercise plan, forget it.
It's not possible. The truth is you will never be perfect. Life will never be perfect. Do you expect yourself to be perfect in maintaining an exercise plan?

Perfectionism is an illusion, like a mirage in the desert. You'll never reach it because it doesn't exist.

Comparisons

What about this statement? *"Others don't have cancer, so it will be harder for me."*

For some, exercising and choosing good foods to eat seems effortless. They may follow the same plan as you do and get totally different results. For you, it is like a recurring trip to the dentist. You know it's going to hurt, and it always seems to cost you in the end.

There will always be that temptation to compare your results to something or someone else. You may even think that no matter what you do, it will never match up to "the competition." Do you tend to compare yourself to others?

Comparing yourself to others and/or your past is a losing battle. The only competition you have is yourself. Progress, no matter how slow, is success.

Expectations

If your expectations are too high, you will set yourself up for failure. In some cases, ER sets in before you even get started. Set incremental goals that take your current health status into account. Learn to manage your time more effectively within your lifestyle changes and start by making your health goals the top priority. Remember – just do the best you can.

Setting expectations too high is self-defeating. Set realistic and attainable goals to measure your progress.

Recognizing your emotions is one thing; managing them is another. Why do most fail at exercise? Why do most people feel lousy in general? For them, the seas are too rough. Calm your mind and the rest with follow.

9
Calming Seas

Restless Minds - Quiet Times

Cancer will make you prioritize your life. Some things don't mean as much as they used to, and others mean so much more. However, the temptation to get back into a busy lifestyle can still nag at you. The first thing you must do to thrive is to develop a proper mindset. With or without cancer, managing emotions plays a vital role in exercise, eating habits and in life.

Emotional Management

So what is the solution to a fast-paced life, negative behaviors, a lack of exercise and/or poor eating habits? Emotional management (EM). EM is how you manage your emotions each day.

If you do not take care of yourself physically and protect yourself emotionally, your energy will be zapped. Stress and reduced emotional strength could weaken your immune system, which often leads to colds or worse. The situation with my mother described earlier in this book is a perfect example of the effects of neglect.

One of the main reasons people are overweight, full of sickness and drained of energy is mismanagement of their emotions.

Restless Minds

Restless minds can and will induce stress. High stress levels encourage you to eat foods that are tasty, but incredibly unhealthy. People with restless minds can be short-sighted, too. People who are short-sighted will go out of their way to get something to eat for taste rather than for health. How can you find a way to put your mind at rest?

Quiet Times

When was the last time you turned off your cell phone?

When was the last time you had a cup of coffee from your *own* coffee machine? Quiet time means quiet time! If you could give yourself as little as 15 minutes per day for some peace and quiet, many of your eating behaviors would change. A busy, restless mind will only hinder your present condition, not help it. Calm the inside waters and the rest of the journey will enjoy smoother sailing.

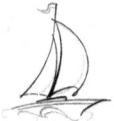

Wind for Your Sails

The **"INSIDE-OUT"** concept takes a look at your exercise and eating behaviors through a cognitive awareness approach. It deals with your motives, desires, and beliefs toward exercise and food. If you want to change attitudes and habits toward fitness and diet for the long haul, you will have to dig deep into *why* you feel the way you do about them.

It will not be pleasant and it will take hard work. The real question is, how important is feeling better to you? And, are you at the point in your life where *there are no more options,* except to move forward?

The key to creating and maintaining the habits of good health is to keep the "big picture" in mind. Be consistent in your exercise routines, no matter if it is just once a week. Incorporate some fun activities in your program and always strive for a quality workout instead of focusing on unrealistic expectations.

It's time to get started; stop resisting it! Listen to your heart - it's telling you how much you really want to feel better. Use the headwinds of hope to propel you toward your goals.

The natural progression is first to learn to cope with the sudden, life-changing experience of cancer.
Next, you must find a way move on, even if the best you can do is to just float along with the current.

The key is learning to consciously carry on. If you start to get some exercise and focus on eating better, who knows? The idea is to take that first step forward, then another and another. What do you have to lose? Find the strength, be the captain of your sailboat and say, "Let's go cruising!"

Part III

Cruising

Survive:
To carry on
To persist
To cope

10
Drifting

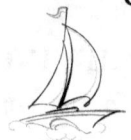

Coping

Most people wait until something of some value is threatened before they will change a lifestyle behavior. Getting healthy is no different. It seems as though the words "heart attack," "stroke," "diabetes" or "cancer" have to come out of the doctor's mouth before you finally understand that it's time to take better care of yourself.

Cancer survivors are different. With other medical conditions, doctors often make suggestions on how to improve your physical health. With cancer, doctors don't always say things like:

"Walk three times a week, stretch and eat less fattening food. This approach will lower your chances of a recurrence and build up your immune system."
In truth, the doctors always should offer this advice, but they often don't.

There are as many ways of coping with cancer as there are cancer patients. For most, numbness takes over the body. You just feel like you're drifting by in life, hoping the news and the pain will go away like a bad dream. Unfortunately, they do not. So, here is your situation; either you are adrift or you make an effort and steadily move forward.

It takes a lot of energy to go in a certain direction, but in the beginning, all you want to do is survive. Getting some exercise and eating the right foods can get you beyond the mindset of bare survival.

Nothing is worse than drifting aimlessly in life. Through exercise, you will have more control over the winds that could blow your life off course. Maybe it's just a psychological crutch, but even if it is only that, it still helps you steadily move forward and carry on.

11
Steady as She Goes

Carrying On

Boats do not operate like cars. You turn the steering wheel of a boat ten times and it only feels like you've moved a foot. However, once you're moving, it's steady as she goes. Somehow, some way, you need to turn your wheels. At some point, you have to decide either to allow cancer to defeat you or to carry on.

You have to find the strength somewhere to get the boat moving again. Eating a healthier diet will give you instant energy to help propel you through the day. If you can muster up enough strength to walk a little, this will get the currents flowing inside. Once you do, you will notice that you have better circulation and more oxygen to your brain, allowing you to think and feel better.

Getting out of shape or getting in better condition is not just physical! Manage your mind and the course will follow.

Greg Ryan

12
Sailing Winds

Big Picture

The key to being motivated is to keep your eye on the horizon. If you don't, the details will become too much headwind to handle. Let the wind behind your sail allow you to *just move forward*; don't worry too much about the rest.

"Big picture" thinking focuses on internal health issues such as lowering your blood pressure, body fat, and cholesterol levels, as well as achieving higher energy levels and a quiet mind.

No Magic Formulas

There are parts to any exercise program that will work. Yet, anything promising fast results is usually too good to be true and will set you up for disappointment. There are no magic formulas to getting healthier, no matter what someone or some product promises you.

More is *Not* Better

If you walk for 20 minutes and burn a certain number of calories, then logic says that if you walk 40 minutes, you will burn twice as many calories and be in better shape. But when you're getting started, a 40-minute walk could seem like a cross-country hike.

Don't put obstacles in your way by expecting too much of yourself in the beginning. If you can truly commit to only a 10 minute walk on a regular basis, that's real progress. Doing a little bit goes a long way, so more is not always better.

Exercise *Smarter*, not Harder

A more demanding workout is not the answer to better results, but exercising effectively and efficiently is. *It's important to incorporate all areas of fitness into a program:* stretching for flexibility, a cardiovascular workout, strength training and balanced eating habits.

Being effective is really important. Energy and emotional management are the keys to being effective. People who understand their own bodies and the proper balance of exercise and eating seem to do less than anyone else and still achieve better results. They've learned the smart way to exercise doesn't have to be so hard.

Emotional Health

More important than waistline measurements or scale readings, developing an effective fitness habit changes you on a deeper level. It builds self-esteem, confidence and discipline. Money can't buy these benefits, nor can you live successfully without them.

Internal vs. External Goals

Internal results come in the form of better vital signs such as lower blood pressure, decreased body fats, lower cholesterol or triglyceride levels, and higher energy levels. Have these as your top priorities, and the other fitness goals will seem to take care of themselves.

More people will stick with a fitness program if they focus on the emotional and internal results more than the external benefits. Also, most people that eat a fairly healthy diet tend to see those desired results happen more quickly.

If you know the basic ins and outs of eating for improved health, you can experience much smoother sailing.

13
Sea Food

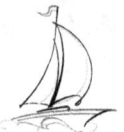

Whether you have cancer or not, two important components to any fitness program are the right map to guide you and a proper perspective on the foods you eat.

The Right Map

The right map has three elements: a good overall mindset, sound eating guidelines and an overall exercise prescription. No matter who you are and how you vary them, all three must be included in your program or you will not reach your goal of long-term success.

Food Perspectives

Eating a healthy diet is about common sense, managing emotions and perseverance.

No matter how you add up the numbers or subtract the fat amounts, it's still the same result: calories taken *in* versus calories burned *out*. It's that simple!

Controlling your calories in and out requires discipline. The unfortunate thing is you can't easily see the internal effects of your poor eating habits.

In your mind, you downplay the importance of following through by only thinking of the immediate gratification that the meal can bring. You need to be more conscious of the effect of what you're putting in your body.

Mindful Eating

It would be nice if someone else told you when and what to eat. Unfortunately, you can't deny that every choice is yours. Conscientious eating requires taking responsibility for your food choices. It also requires you to take the emotions out of the decision process.

Emotional Eating

Most of your eating habits have an underlying emotional attachment to them. Knee-jerk reactions to circumstances point you toward food for emotional security. In most cases, you go for taste. You usually choose taste over your health because of your lifestyle. You're too busy to fix a good meal...or too lazy!

Lifestyle Eating

Eating habits are in some way dictated by your lifestyle. You eat what, where and when you can, often on the go. This is not good! Getting control of your lifestyle will curb your negative food habits.

Attitudes of Eating

When trying to maintain a balanced and sensible eating plan, there are a few things to remember that you will not find in a recipe, diet book or classroom. They are the five P's of eating; perspectives, patterns, provocations, portions and planning.

Perspectives on Eating

If you eat just because you're overly hungry, then your choice of foods will be more for taste rather than for health.
Most of us eat because it is a necessity to live and maintain energy.

If you had the attitude that food was fuel, would that change what you eat? Would you be more inclined to make better choices? Your attitude toward food is very important! Your self-worth, security, and comfort in life are not derived from food. They come from deeper within. Recognize that food is fuel, not an anti-depressant.

Eating Patterns

You tend to eat at the same time, gobble up the same food types, and in most cases, you take in roughly the same amount of food on a weekly basis. It is really important to incorporate a variety of foods in your daily eating program. This change in your eating patterns will help your body adapt to the increase in activity and the decrease in calories.

Provocations to Eat

If you plan ahead, you may not have to rely on the fast food industry for your meals. If you think about it, many times your eating habits are emotional reactions to magazine, billboard or TV advertisements.

Also, don't shop for groceries on an empty stomach. Ice cream, chips and soft drinks almost literally call to you from the aisles when you're hungry. It's important to think about and recognize those external cues that cause you to eat unhealthy foods.

Portion Sizes

Being aware of how much you eat at one time is very important. Even though pasta is a healthy food type, the extra one or two hundred calories a few times a week adds up. Learn to push the plate away. Calories add up, so think about what you're eating, eat more slowly and choose smaller portions.

Develop a Plan

It boils down to time management. If you have better, healthier choices in the refrigerator, you will likely eat the foods you have on hand.

When healthy foods are unavailable, it's easier to get to the cookies in the pantry, the pizza parlor, or the fast food restaurant for immediate gratification. If you pre-plan your week of eating, it will be easier to make better choices.

Behavior Changes

You can say what you want to about the abrasive approach of a self-help guru like Dr. Phil, but don't criticize the thinking behind it; you have to change your behaviors in order to change your life. It makes a lot of sense, doesn't it?

You can't escape the fact that eating patterns are for some reason lodged in your brain. Like Dr. Phil says, until you *"get real"* with them and recognize that you need to change, you're only kidding yourself. This is especially true with regard to your eating habits.

Numbers Don't Lie

If you want to feel better and have more energy, you have to consciously monitor your portions of food. The number of calories does add up, whether the foods are good or bad for you.

What we need to do as a country and as individuals is get back to the basics of healthy eating. Once you understand those basics, it's not a complicated process.

"Less" Can Mean More

"Well, if there is less fat, then I can eat twice the amount and get away with it." Have you ever thought about food this way? Unfortunately, if you don't take into con-sideration the calories of the extra food you're eating, the low-fat alternatives are just as dangerous as the high-fat choices.

Empty Calories

One thing you may not realize is some fats can be used as good fuel. When taken out of the food, the nutritional value can be reduced. Foods with little or no nutritional value, such as low-fat cookies or soft drinks, are simply empty calories.

No Permission Slips

Your food habits are not entirely behavioral.

There are some things inside the body that encourage you to eat in unhealthy ways. Have you ever wondered why you seem to crave something sweet at certain times of the day or night? Or do you ever get sleepy around mid-morning or afternoon? This may have something to do with blood sugar levels in the body. When your sugar levels drop, your body is looking for quick fixes like candy, snack foods, sodas and other simple carbohydrates. Just because your body sends you a signal, this is not a "permission slip" to eat unhealthy foods.

Below are some eating habits that cause your body to send those tempting signals:

Simple Carbohydrates

Foods high in simple carbohydrates like pasta, white breads, potatoes, candy, chips and soft drinks can give you sugar "highs." Without proteins to balance your food intake, these simple foods that quickly turn into sugar in your body can cause "sugar drop," draining you of energy and causing cravings for more sugary foods.

Portions

Large portions of food also may cause sugar highs and crashes. Be aware of the amounts of food you eat at one time. Your body also has to expend a lot more energy to digest larger amounts of food, which robs you of energy you could use for other purposes.

Timing

If you allow too much time between meals, you face a sugar low, which tempts you to binge. When your blood sugar drops, the natural tendency is to grab lots of something tasty, like chips, candy or even a high-fat, sugary coffee-house beverage.

Learn what are the red-flag foods and drinks and work to avoid them. A good attitude is:

PROPER PLANNING PREVENTS POOR PERFORMANCE!

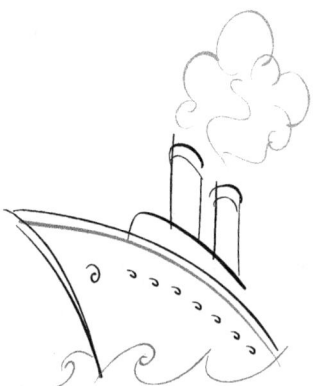

14
Watch Out for Mines

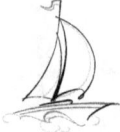

Knowing Where They Are

It doesn't matter what you're going through or what your goals are for getting in better shape. You have to learn where the mines are in your eating habits to avoid them. Here are a few general "diet bombs":

Soft Drinks

Sodas act like a beacon for calories. Diet or otherwise, it doesn't matter; high-calorie simple carbohydrates and fatty foods go hand-in-hand with soft drinks. In the long run, ignoring this fact will be very detrimental to your efforts to feel better, improve your circulation or build up your immune system.

Additives and Preservatives

If at all possible, reduce the amount of foods with additives and preservatives in your eating plan. Foods with high levels of unnatural preservatives clog the system. Natural, organic or whole foods are best.

White vs. Wheat

White rice, bread or potatoes are more easily converted into sugar in the body and can make you sluggish. Try to cut down on these types of food. You will notice the difference almost immediately.

Other Simple Carbohydrates

Whether they are a physiological need of the body or an emotional addiction, simple carbohydrates are quickly digested and converted to sugar in the blood stream. Simple carbohydrates include candy, chips, cakes and cookies, as well the sodas discussed above.

On the other hand, complex carbohydrates, such as high-fiber breads, pasta, sweet potatoes and brown rice, are more slowly and evenly digested. Eating these foods reduces the chances of sugar highs and lows, encourages the absorption of necessary nutrients and leads to better intestinal health.

Non-fat Foods

High-fat foods that have been altered with fat-free alternatives tend to have extra salt and sugar, which adds empty, non-nutritious calories. Be careful of manufacturer's claims and read labels – don't eat these "non-fat" foods in large quantities. Remember, foods that are normally loaded with calories but are now altered to be "low-calorie" can be deceiving. Fat-free and low-sugar additives can also have a negative impact on your digestive system, causing unwanted affects on your stomach or bowels.

Night time and Off-time Feeding

Be careful of eating late into the evening hours. The digestive process takes extra energy, robbing your body of the ability to rest efficiently.

Also, be aware of and resist the urge to eat when you are bored.

Eating out of boredom instead of a real nutritional need only adds unnecessary calories to your diet. Drink water, chew gum or occupy your mind with other distractions instead of eating to pass the time.

Less Is *Not* Best

Falling into the trap of eating less in order to avoid gaining weight is a big mistake. The body goes into a protection mode and even slows down its metabolism. Low blood sugar and a low metabolism equal low energy.

All or Nothing

If you decide that you can only win at your diet if you never eat ice cream again, you will surely fail.

Having an "all or nothing" attitude will drive you nuts. The need to be "perfect" can be a disease of the mind. Eating and exercise is a balancing act. If you allow yourself the occasional treat *in moderation*, you will have better success in sticking with a healthy diet and exercise routine.

Healthy Eating Tips:

- ❖ Never shop for food when hungry.
- ❖ Eat a balanced plate of food, including protein, complex carbohydrates and fruits or vegetables with each meal.
- ❖ Lower the amounts of food eaten later at night.
- ❖ Lower the amount of white-flour foods, additives and preservatives.
- ❖ Sit while you eat.
- ❖ Eat with your opposite hand.
- ❖ Don't allow more than four hours between snacks or meals.
- ❖ Always eat breakfast.
- ❖ Put variety into your diet and eating patterns.
- ❖ Drink lots of fluids, but avoid sodas.
- ❖ Keep a food diary to become more aware of what and when you eat.
- ❖ Eat slowly and only until you are comfortable.
- ❖ Lower the amounts of caffeine and alcohol.
- ❖ Vary the sources and amounts of your calories daily.

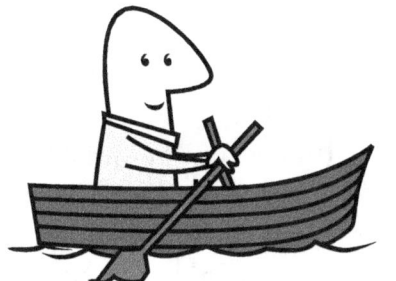

15
Row, Row, Row your Boat

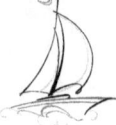

Back to Basics

If you keep the basics in mind, exercise and healthy eating are not that difficult. Do you know how much food you eat on a daily basis? How about the total calories you consume each day? Here are the basic numbers when determining total calories and fat grams.

<u>Facts & Figures</u>

1 gram of Fat = 9 calories
1 gram of Protein = 4 calories
1 gram of Carbohydrates = 4 calories

<u>Fat % per Serving Formula</u>

1. Fat grams x 9 = total fat calories.
2. Fat calories / total calories = fat %
3. Fat % Goal – Less than 30 % per serving.

Reading Labels

Take the time to read about what you are eating. Commercially-packaged foods must be labeled and list most if not all of their ingredients, along with other nutritional data. You can usually tell in the first few listed ingredients if the food is natural or full of preservatives and artificial ingredients.

Emotions and Eating

Eating patterns often have something to do with an underlying emotion. Emotions do not distinguish between good and bad foods. They just want to be comforted and food is a great security blanket! Be aware of your emotions as a possible source of cravings.

Lifestyle, Genetics and Eating

You are going to have to change your lifestyle if you want to change your eating habits. Be mindful of when, why and what you eat.

Some people can afford to eat more due to a naturally high metabolism. Be careful - aging and inactivity lower metabolic rates.

16
Go with the Current

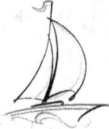

Keep it Simple!

Keep things simple and go with the flow. Don't try to invent some new way of doing things. First, remember the basic guidelines of consistent exercise and a healthy diet. A good exercise and fitness protocol to follow is from the **American College of Sports Medicine.**

A.C.S.M. guidelines

The American College of Sports Medicine (A.C.S.M.) suggests weekly workout guidelines for cardiovascular, strength and flexibility training. These guidelines are the focus of this chapter.

While exercise and eating guidelines are based on good scientific principles, they do not necessarily agree with human nature or common sense.

Recent history tells us that we are better off encouraging the people who are willing to include exercise in their daily lives than forcing guidelines on the majority of those who want to fight the inevitable.

In the end, keeping things simple, supportive and selective will change the heart as well as the body.

Greg Ryan

Matters of the Heart

Cardiovascular training means exercising the heart by maintaining an elevated heart rate for a specific amount of time. Sorry, walking on the golf course or just taking the stairs every day doesn't cut it. Sure, those extra activities burn calories, but they don't have the same strengthening affect on your cardiovascular system.

Heart Rate Zones (THR)

In my experience, this is one of the most under-utilized measuring tools in most exercise programs. With this tool, you can learn to work smarter, not necessarily harder.

In order to lose weight, drop blood pressure or lose body fat, you must exercise within your heart rate zone for a certain amount of time and at a certain rate of intensity, several times during the week. The heart rate formula that calculates your cardiovascular zone is: 220 – age x (60-85%) = Target Heart Rate.

Frequency

A.C.S.M. recommends you try to exercise your heart three to five times in seven days.

Duration

A.C.S.M. suggests that you achieve 20 - 40 minutes within your heart rate zone each workout. Please just start out at five minutes and move up to the goal. Do not get discouraged if you can't reach your goal in the beginning.

Practice Flexibility

Flexibility training means stretching the joints, tendons and muscles to the point of stress. This is by far the most neglected part of any workout program. Why? It can hurt, there is no instant gratification and it takes a little extra time. So what?

Types of Stretching

There are two different types of flexibility stretches: ballistic and static. Ballistic stretching involves putting the joints and muscles through a bouncing type of stretch.

This type of stretch is not recommended. The other type is called static stretching. This type is where you stretch a particular muscle for a length of time in slow movements.

When to Stretch

There is some confusion in the workout community as to when to stretch. You would think you would want to stretch before you workout to warm up and you are right! However, you want to stretch even more *after* your workout. This helps the rebuilding process of muscles and joints.

How Often?

Stretching, if done correctly, should be performed many times during the week. If you don't know how to stretch or which stretches are best, there are charts available that demonstrate the proper forms for stretching. If flexibility training is neglected, your workout will not be as effective and could possibly result in negative results.

The Strong Do Survive

The definition of obesity is when your body fat level is thirty percent or more of your total body weight.

Strength training and muscle conditioning decreases those levels considerably by burning calories, increasing muscle mass and raising metabolic rates. Strength training also helps to increase circulation and bone strength, lower triglyceride levels, and improve your posture. There are general rules you should follow when weight training. These may vary depending upon age or if you are in a specific sport, but in general, the following guidelines apply:

Frequency

For general conditioning, two to three times in a seven-day period is sufficient. The main rule is leave at least one day between similar workouts. Body muscles, unlike the heart muscle, need time to recuperate.

Duration

Generally speaking, a weight training session of 30 to 40 minutes is adequate. A longer workout means you're probably only working harder, not smarter.

Recuperation

When it comes to strength training, more is not better! It goes against logic, but muscles are not building during your workout. They grow while they recuperate and rest. This is why sleep, good nutrition and a balanced program are important. Unfortunately, many people learn this lesson the hard way and end up hurting themselves. If you are efficient during your workouts, then your body will respond in more positive way. Eighty percent of those currently exercising don't follow a good set of guidelines.

A.C.S.M. Guidelines

Cardiovascular Training (Heart)
Time: 3-5 times a week
Duration: 20- 40 minutes
Intensity: 220 –age x (60-85%) =
             Target Heart Zone
Flexibility Training (Joints)
Time: Daily

Duration:	10 minutes
Intensity:	No bouncing
	Ten to twenty-second count

Strength Training (Skeletal Muscles)

Time:	2-3 times a week
Duration:	20-40 minutes
Intensity:	Strength: 8-12 repetitions
	Endurance: 10-15 repetitions

Support and Accountability

All of these guidelines are important, but if you don't have a support or accountability system in place, you will not follow through.

A good support team around you factors heavily into your success. Seek out those family members or friends that are positive and encouraging about your health goals.

It may be possible to survive for a while without some form of accountability, but you will not thrive without taking responsibility for your health. No one can make decisions or do the work for you. Your success is up to you and you alone.

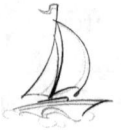

Wind for Your Sails

Drifting in life may be the only thing you can do at first. Somehow, some way, learn to carry on. A busy life and expensive gadgets make your eating habits more complicated – learn to simplify your life. Just because it says "low-fat" doesn't mean it's better for you. Eating is an emotional as well as a physical response. You have to work on the feelings, too.

While guidelines are necessary, try not to get bogged down with the details. Decide to make exercise and eating a healthy diet the priorities in your life. Don't get discouraged, even if the results don't always meet your expectations.

Eating right has a lot to do with how you look at food, how much you eat and what you eat. Use common sense and listen to your body. Be aware of red flags.

Think about when, why and what you're eating, before you eat. Determine whether you have eating patterns. The patterns may be related to lifestyle, emotions, physical concerns, or all the above. Pre-planning meals can avoid a lot of the poor eating decisions. Learn to push yourself away from the table.

Keep it simple, stick to the basics, and you will have a better chance of staying with the program. Most importantly, don't be afraid to ask for help and support. A positive environment produces positive results.

Despite your experience with cancer, the right perspectives on food and a "keep it simple" approach to exercise will build energy, confidence, strong bones and a better quality of life.

Part IV

Ship Mates

"Your success and future may depend on your ability to face your fears and ask for help."

Greg Ryan

17
Buoys

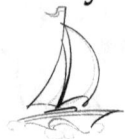

The A Factor

Buoys are markers or guides for big ships. As you continue to get healthier you need markers to guide you, too. One thing that will ensure your direction is to get good support around you. Accepting that fact, asking for assistance and taking the first steps toward better health by having someone hold you accountable are all key factors. You could call these steps *"The A Factor."*

In other words, personal accountability and responsibility are definitely required.

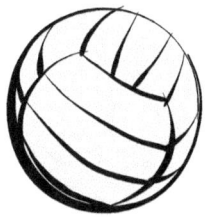

*Don't worry, Wilson...I'll do all the paddling. You
just hang on.*

Chuck Noland
"Cast Away"

18
Your "Wilson"

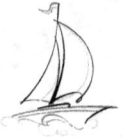

Have you ever felt like saying to your doctor?

Don't you dare say to me, "There's nothing we can do." My circumstances have nothing to do with "we". I have lived my life rowing upstream and if you think I am going to stop paddling now and give up, forget it.

I know, you're going to give me some brochures for support and send me on my way; leaving me to drift on the depressed waves of life. Sorry, but surviving is just not good enough. As a far as I'm concern, you might as well sail on down the hall to some other poor vessel and try to sell them a ticket to no where because I'm not buying.

Denial, no; I know what the difference is between reality and wishful thinking.
I accept the former, but that does not mean I have to stop living, does it?

It is important to reiterate the impact of having a person around you to whom you can talk about your desires to feel better through exercise and healthy foods. We all need a "Wilson" around us who we can use as a sounding board for our ideas, emotions and fears.

As silly as it sounds, if the character of Chuck Noland in the movie "Cast Away" didn't have Wilson (the volleyball) there to talk to on that island, he would have lost hope and died. Silly? Yes, but life-saving, too.

The "A" Team

Creating the "A" Team is about asking for support, getting encouragement and being held accountable. A doctor, an account-ability partner or an exercise trainer are all good advisors to have on your "A" Team.

Doctor

Make sure you get regular checkups. Let the doctor know that you are exercising and eating a more healthy diet.

Partnerships

Tell someone close to you what you are doing. Let them in on your goals and desires. Give them permission to hold you accountable toward achieving your goals.

Trainers

If need be, hire a personal trainer to help guide and motivate you. This will save you time and effort in the long run, and give you much needed encouragement.

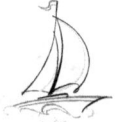

Wind for Your Sails

First, take responsibility for your health. Being a victim will not get you off the couch; being grateful will. None of us are promised tomorrow, no matter what cards have been dealt our way. Read the book, "Happiness is a Choice," by Barry Neil Kaufman.

And second, don't be afraid to ask for help. Find a friend in a "Wilson" out there to talk to, help you and guide you through this tough time.

Keep your doctor informed, find an accountability partner and hire a trainer, if necessary. Whatever you do, get off the couch, put your engine in gear and get moving. You don't want to just survive--you really want to thrive, don't you?

Part V

Full Throttle

THRIVE:
To make steady progress
To flourish

19
Full Steam Ahead

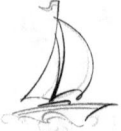

Flourishing

It may take a boat a while to get up to full steam, but once it does, watch it go! Life after cancer can have the same momentum, once you get moving. Your life can flourish and blossom, but only if you take care of it.

Your Best Offense

Let's face the facts: exercise, just like life, will never be as perfect as you would like. Your past failures with diets and fitness programs have no bearing on your future, and there will never be a more ideal time than now to start. Your best offense is to *just move it!*

Most of you will think your way into bad health. You will talk yourself out of exercise, make excuses and just be lazy.

Your best bet is to work to prevent bad health by having a forward-thinking attitude. In other words, take a proactive and preventative approach to better health; don't just react to what life sends your way.

Another thing to avoid is being overwhelmed. Just remember: it's more about your will to improve than numbers on a chart.

Your Worst Defense

The worst thing you can do is to do ***nothing***. Yes, cancer at first can and will be paralyzing. But, sooner or later you have to start up your engine and press on the throttle.

To turn around a well-known phrase, sometime the worst defense is a weak (or no) offense. Make a decision, get help, and do whatever it takes to get out on the waters of life.

20
Over the Bounty Waves

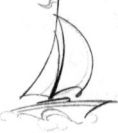

Ok, I want to feel better and am willing to get off the couch. But I have a few questions:

Does having had cancer limit me in exercising?

When do I start?

Where do I begin?

What do I do?

How do I know what the future holds?

Outer Limits

Having had cancer may limit you in certain ways. Talk to your doctor first for advice on how to determine your limitations. If he/she says it's ok, then start **at your own pace**. Guidelines are great, but not a must.

Your energy level in the beginning will determine your choice of activity and the amount of effort you wish to make.

When to Start

Nothing is more enjoyable than to skip over the top of the waves with the wind at your back. But how do you get to that point? You have to have the will to start, no matter where your boat is docked.

When should you start exercising? Even if you don't want to begin, you should start as soon as you can, preferably within a month of leaving the hospital. This will require some faith, a little hope and possibly some help from others. Getting started is just as important for your self-confidence as it is for your health.

Where to Begin

Start by just taking a short walk. Your energy level will determine the amount of activity. Ask someone to go with you if that helps. If you're worried about your pride, lose it. If you are lazy, push through it. If you are resentful, get over it. Don't let cancer convince you that you can't do something. Make the decision to start, find the strength that is within you, and *just do it*.

What to Do

The Heart

Walking gets your blood circulating, builds up the antibodies in the blood, and even helps your brain function better. Ride a stationary bike, try swimming or put on some music at home and dance - anything to get the blood flowing again.

The Joints

Stretching is another good thing to start doing right away. In addition to walking, stretching the joints improves your circulation, strengthens tendons and helps prevent stiffness. It's easy to go at your own pace and doesn't require expensive clothes or equipment.

The Muscles

Eventually, it is important for you to start doing some exercises that strengthen your muscles, especially those in your legs, chest and back. It may take some time to get to this point, but stronger muscles really help to boost the immune system, perform everyday activities and raise confidence levels.

Your Future

It's true that you don't know what the future holds. Experiencing cancer puts a whole new perspective on life, or at least it should. Exercise and eating well may not add another day, but what if it could? What if it gave you a better quality of life?

If you want to sail, you must first want to live. If you want to live, you have to get off the dock. Paddle first, get the wind behind you, and before you know it, you will be sailing.

Be a sailor!

21
Fellow Sailors

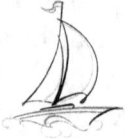

Bill (age 55)

I didn't deserve this, I thought, when I first heard I had prostate cancer. Life was going great. Grandkids were growing. I was just getting ready to retire, and I thought my health was doing ok.

Our family maybe didn't have the best eating habits, but the doctor said my vital signs were within reason. What caused the cancer? I don't know. I don't really care at this point. I do care, however, about sticking around to see my grandkids grow up. You bet - I <u>will</u> take better care of myself now.

Beth (age 58)

I knew breast cancer ran in our family, but I didn't want to think about it happening to me. Denial? Maybe. However, when it did, life stood still. Why me? What do I do now?
Where does my future lie? All questions I had no answer to.

What made me even more upset was I took care of myself. I ate right, I exercised and never had a cold. It didn't make any sense. One day, I just said, "enough is enough. Suck it up, be grateful and move ahead the best you can."

Thank God for my family and friends. Thank God for not looking back.

Jim (age 65)

I stopped smoking 20 years ago. Why now? I thought I could be past the point of cancer. I don't get it, but I must accept it. Do I? Yes, but I'm not giving up. Never was a quitter and I'm not going to start now.

Up until now I was never a regular exerciser, either, but I am now. Too bad it took losing some lung to get the point.

Kathy (age 48)

The doctor says "two years." I say, "we'll see." Am I angry? I was at first.
Now I just realize it's a waste of energy and time to be mad or resentful.

I jumped out of an airplane not too long ago. They say if you want to soar like eagles, you have to jump out of your plane. So I did. Was I scared? I was more scared of dying with regrets than parachuting. Am I scared of my future? No. In some strange way, cancer has been the best thing for me and my life.

I just wish I could explain to you what it's like to live your life everyday like you were dying. I don't wish cancer on anyone, but I do wish you understood how precious and short life really is.

A good team is one that provides quality support, supplies honest encouragement, and requires personal responsibility.

Greg Ryan

22
Sail on, Sailor

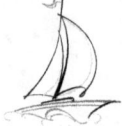

Sail On

In 2005, Tim McGraw wrote a country song called, *"Live Like You Were Dying."* It was named the most inspiring song of the year. The song was dedicated to Tim's father, Tug McGraw, the famous baseball player.

As a person who has gone through a bout with cancer, this song may not have the same meaning to you as it would to others. For you, the words of the song may have a deep and personal effect.

For the rest of us, life should not be taken for granted. If we are fortunate enough to have tomorrow, let's be the healthiest and happiest we can. But, you already know this, don't you?

Hopefully, you don't just want to survive, you want to thrive. I used exercising and eating well to better my life; I encourage you to do the same. They both saved my life and they could do the same for you. This doesn't have to be the beginning of the end, but instead, an invitation to go sailing on the sea of a healthier, more vibrant life. Never settle for less when you can have more and definitely never allow some doctor in a lab coat tell you, *"Sorry, there is nothing we can do."*

Do you want to flourish? Do it by being more active. Even though he's just a fictional character, the inspirational Chuck Noland never stopped believing. He chose to live, never to forget about the next tide that came in. When you feel like giving up, just think about how Chuck described his will to go on:

"And that's when this feeling came over me like a warm blanket. I knew, somehow, that I had to stay alive. Somehow. I had to keep breathing. Even though there was no reason to hope. And all my logic said that I would never see this place again. So that's what I did. I stayed alive. I kept breathing. And one day my logic was proven all wrong because the tide came in, and gave me a sail.

And I know what I have to do now. I gotta keep breathing. Because, tomorrow, the sun will rise. Who knows what the tide could bring?"

My Own Voyage

In my twenty years of helping people feel better through exercise and eating well, I have yet to find someone who can prove to me that this process of taking care of your health has any negative side effects.

Emotional Side Effects

When I first was introduced to exercise and healthy eating, I began each day with a glimmer of hope - hope that I could do something positive with my life through exercise, hope that I could help someone else through my own experiences, and hope that someday I could give back to others what life has giving to me. All I had was hope.

Today, there are still times I don't feel like getting off of the couch and going for a walk, saying no to some apple pie or working to correct bad habits.

But it's that hope for the future that keeps me going, even if it's just for one more day. My father taught me to work hard, have faith, and treat others with respect. It was easy for him to say, but not so easy for me to follow.
Treating others kindly was much easier than having faith in me.

Life was scary for me growing up. I was afraid of not meeting the expectations of those around me. I didn't know what direction to take in life or what advice to follow. When I first stepped into a health club, it was equally as frightening.

I had two friends who exercised with me on a regular basis. The confidence they had in me started to positively affect my attitude and wear down my fear of failure. After a while, I noticed those fears I had about myself slowly began to disappear.

Then one day, it dawned on me. Somewhere down deep inside, I believed I was doing something good. I suddenly knew that with the advice of my father, having realistic expectations, and keeping a one-day-at-a-time attitude, I could change.
With a little bit of hope, mixed in with some faith, I knew I could really make things happen. The more I thought about the good I was doing for myself, the more I believed in me.

As I developed more confidence, I started to realize how important it was for this change to come from the inside out. Looking better, having more energy and getting physically stronger were great things to experience, but I was most grateful for the changes in my heart and in my spirit.

I felt better about myself. I had purpose and I was doing something positive. That heartfelt motivation became the glue that has kept me going for all these years. No matter what you do in life, if you have purpose, and if it is good for others, life will be rewarding. Your *motives* must come from within. Most importantly, I have never forgotten where I started, what I have had to go through and where I am going. It all began for me with a little bit of *hope*.

Physical Side Effects

I could fill another book on the positive side effects of exercise. But, what about those who have had cancer?

I'm not a doctor. I'm just a person who uses common sense, personal experience, exercise, healthy eating and the power of hope to help others.

Both medical studies and common sense can show you how regular exercise builds up immune systems, improves circulation, strengthens bones, and keeps joints from freezing up. Many more studies have proven the benefits of a healthy diet for improving both the quality and duration of life.

Now, don't you think a cancer survivor could benefit from exercise and healthy eating? Just think of the potential. I'm not saying that exercise and eating better can cure all, but what if they could help you feel better, give you more energy and increase your confidence? My hope and purpose for this book is to let you know that there is life after cancer.

Sail on, Sailor!

Live Like You Were Dying
by Tim McGraw

He said I was in my early forties,
With a lot of life before me,
And a moment came that stopped me on a dime.
I spent most of the next days, lookin' at the x-rays,
Talkin' 'bout the options and talkin' 'bout sweet time.
Asked him when it sank in, that this might really be
the real end.
How's it hit ya, when you get that kind of news.
Man what ya do.
And he says,

Chorus:
I went sky divin',
I went rocky mountain climbin',
I went 2.7 seconds on a bull name Fu Manchu.
And I loved deeper,
And I spoke sweeter,
And I gave forgiveness I've been denying,
And he said someday I hope you get the chance,
To live like you were dyin'.

He said I was finally the husband,
That most the time I wasn't.
And I became a friend a friend would like to have.
And all the sudden goin' fishing,
Wasn't such an imposition.
And I went three times that year I lost my dad.
Well I finally read the Good Book,
And I took a good long hard look at what I'd do
If I could do it all again.
And then.

[Chorus]

Like tomorrow was a gift and you've got eternity
To think about what you do with it,
What could you do with it,
What can I do with it,
What would I do with it.

[Chorus]
Sky divin',
I went rocky mountain climbin',
I went 2.7 seconds on a bull name Fu Manchu.
And I loved deeper,
And I spoke sweeter,
And I watched an eagle as it was flyin'.
And he said someday I hope you get the chance,
To live like you were dyin'.

To live like you were dyin'.
To live like you were dyin'.
To live like you were dyin'.
To live like you were dyin'.
Thank You

Thank you for reading, Hope Floats. I wish you all the blessings in the world this coming year. I trust you have retained something of importance in making your health better.

I have a wealth of FREE information on weight loss, fitness, nutrition and bodybuilding.

Website: www.resolutions.bz
Email: greg@resolutions.bz
FREE Fitness Advice
Blogs:
www.resolutionsblog.com
www.reso-care.com
www.gregryanfitness.com

  You Tube Linked in

Check out my entire book collection at

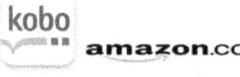 BARNES&NOBLE
BOOKSELLERS